A Brief Guide to Antibody-drug Conjugate

Authored by Alice Brown

Table of Contents

A Brief Guide to Antibody-drug Conjugate 1

Table of Contents 2

Chapter One Introduction 3

Chapter Two Basics about Antibody-drug Conjugate 4

    1.1 Definition 4

    1.2 Main characteristics 4

    1.3 Mechanism of action (MOA) 4

    1.4 Components 5

Chapter Three Challenges for future research development (future prospect) 7

Chapter Four Summary 8

References 9

Chapter One Introduction

If you are fanatic about keeping up with the latest medical trends, then the term **Antibody-drug conjugates** (also called ADCs) shouldn't be foreign to you. Over the past few decades, antibody–drug conjugates have revolutionized the field of cancer chemotherapy. Many experts view it as a more effective method to combat the daunting disease-cancer. Unlike the conventional treatments which will also damage healthy tissues during dose escalation, it intends to target and kill exclusively the cancer cells and thus spares healthy cells.

For this reason, the focused delivery of the cytotoxic agent to the tumor cell is introduced to maximize the anti-tumor effect of ADCs, while at the same time minimizing its normal tissue exposure, potentially bringing an improved therapeutic index.

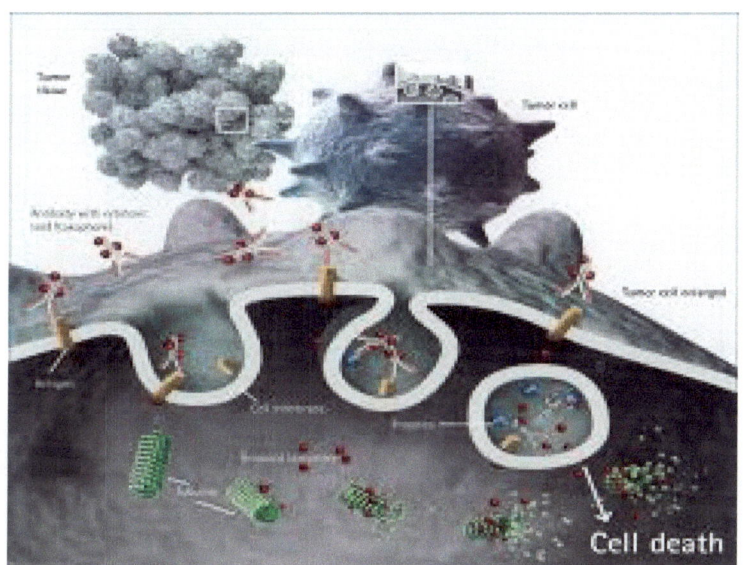

Chapter Two Basics about Antibody-drug Conjugate

1.1 Definition

Antibody-drug conjugates refer to an important class of highly potent biopharmaceutical drugs, specially designed as a targeted therapy for the treatment of cancer. ADCs are virtually complex molecules that are composed of an antibody linked to a biologically active cytotoxic payload or drug.

1.2 Main characteristics

Antibody-drug conjugates are favored by most researchers for its ability of increasing cell-killing potential of mAbs and conferring higher tumor selectivity. Consequently, the tolerability of the drugs is substantially enhanced.

However, a unique characteristic of ADCs, which we must not neglected, is that there is only limited harmful exposure, compared with the conventionally used chemotherapeutic drugs. These so-called armed antibodies selectively dispatch highly potent cytotoxic to cancer cells directly while, at the same time, leaving healthy tissue unaffected. As far as we know, conventional chemotherapy is aimed at eliminating fast-spreading tumor cells. It can, nevertheless, also harm healthy proliferating cells, which definitely will cause undesirable side effects. It is precisely out of consideration for this that ADCs are designed to increase the efficacy of therapy and reduce systemic toxicity.

1.3 Mechanism of action (MOA)

Antibody-drug conjugates are essentially fine examples of bioconjugates and immunoconjugates. It is a three-component system with a potent cytotoxic (anticancer) agent linked to an antibody via a biodegradable linker. A simplified version of its MOA could be like this: the antibody binds to specific markers (namely antigens or receptors) at the surface of the cancer cell. Then the whole antibody-drug conjugate is internalized within the cancer cell, where the linker is degraded and the active drug released accordingly. A curtailed yet vivid graph is presented below for your understanding.

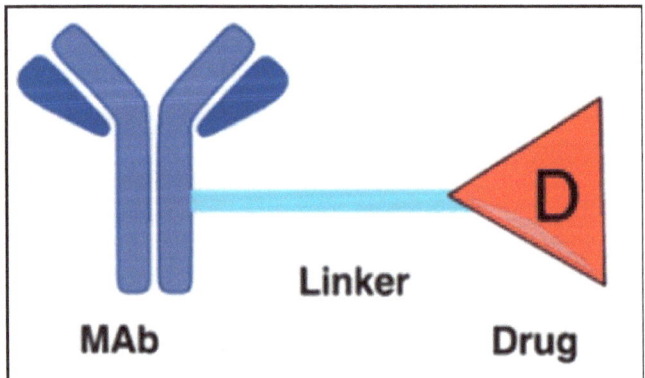

Or the MOA process of ADCs could be more professionally explained in detail as follows: when certain portion of the antibody-drug conjugate is administered intravenously localizes to a tumor and binds to a target antigen on the cell-surface of the tumor cell, the complex will be internalized into the cell. Closely following internalization, the internalized vesicles will fuse with other vesicles and enter the *endosome-lysosome* pathway. In the lysosome, proteases in mild acidic environment digest the monoclonal antibody to release free payloads, which then cross the lysosome membrane to enter the cytoplasm or the nucleus where they bind to the target molecule which, in turn, leads to cell death.

By combining the unique targeting capabilities of monoclonal antibodies with the cancer-killing ability of cytotoxic drugs, antibody-drug conjugates make it possible to sensitively discriminate between healthy and diseased tissue. To put it another way, antibody-drug conjugates, in stark contrast to traditional chemotherapeutic agents, target and attack only the cancer cells so that healthy cells are saved from being severely affected.

1.4 Components

The three components of ADCs are **mAb**, **linker** and **cytotoxin**. All are critical to the efficacy and toxicity of the conjugate. Therefore, it has been a persisting pursuit for researchers to optimize each component and meanwhile enhancing the functionality of the ADC as a whole. Being fully aware of that, let's go deep into each one in the following section.

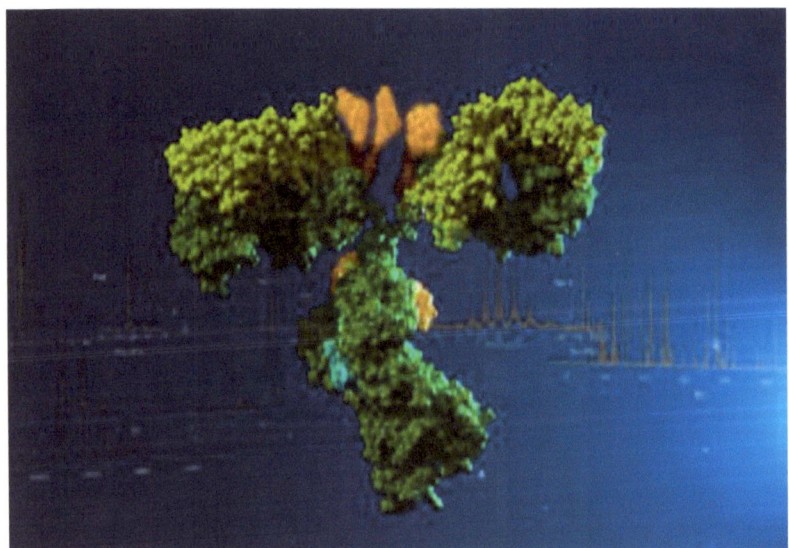

- **Cytotoxic drugs**

There are thousands of cellular toxins from either natural sources or chemical synthesis, but only a very few are proved suitable as components for use in an Antibody-drug Conjugate (ADCs). In the development of early ADCs, researchers used clinically approved chemotherapeutic drugs just because these agents have been already available and their toxicological properties were well known to researchers.

However, the potency these early ADCs and the effect to kill the targeted tumor cells were not that impressive compared with the corresponding unconjugated agents.

To solve this problem, scientists started to look at compounds found to be too toxic when tested as a stand-alone chemotherapeutic agent. But the number of these high potent toxins, generally 100 to 1,000 times more toxic than traditional anticancer agents and are stable, is quite limited.

Among all these used in combination to humanized mAb targeting agents, there are highly potent, biologically active anti-microtubule agents, alkylating agents and DNA minor groove binding agents.

These drugs are biologically active at the ng/Kg level, which helps place them in the most potent class of advanced cancer drugs.

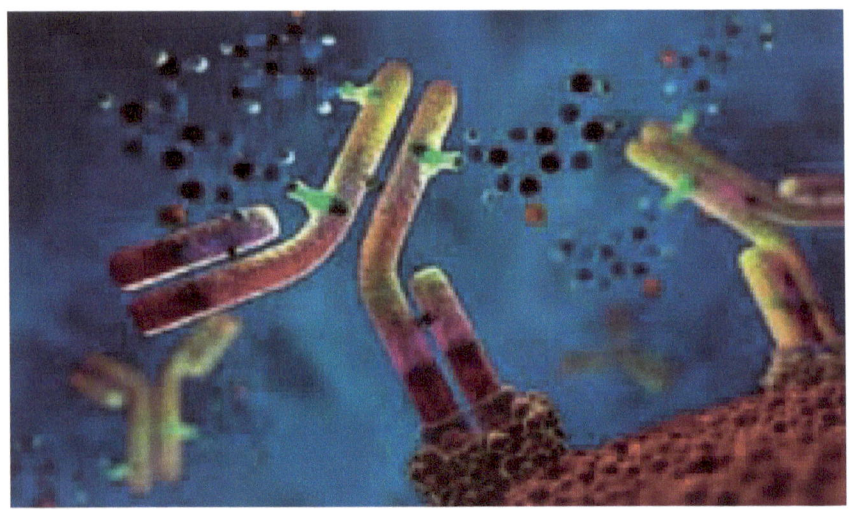

- **Monoclonal Antibodies (mAbs)**

Monoclonal Antibodies are one type of biological therapies to treat diseases, cancer in particular. They first recognize and find specific proteins on cancer cells, and then work in different ways to serve their roles depending on the protein they are targeting. Each monoclonal antibody only recognizes one particular protein. So it won't be strange to see different monoclonal antibodies been made to target different types of cancer. Up till now, there are already a number of mABs available for cancer treatment. Some have gained access to market while newer types are still in clinical trials.

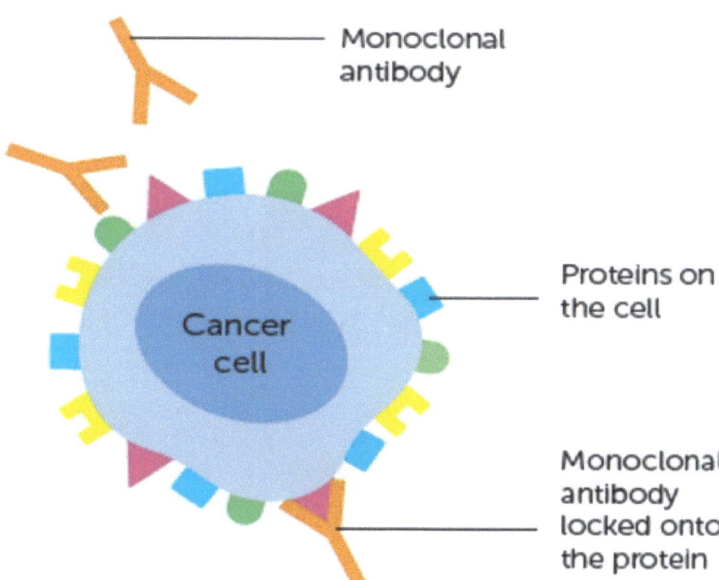

(From Cancer Research UK)

- **Linker**

The linker that connects the cytotoxic drug to the mAb plays a determining role among a string of ADC activities from selectivity, pharmacokinetics, and therapeutic index to overall success of the ADC. These linkers covalently couple the cytotoxic drug to the antibody, together producing an ADC that should be relatively stable in circulation.

Target/MAb
- Exploitable Selectivity
  - High Expression on tumor
  - Limited normal tissue expression
- Limited heterogeneity
- Internalizes following binding
- Conjugation sites (cysteine or lysine) should not impact stability, binding, internalization, pk

Linker
- Stable in circulation
- Selective intracellular release of biologically active drug
  - enzymatic cleavage
  - MAb degradation
- Limited heterogeneity of drug product

Drug
- Highly Potent
- Amenable to modifications that allow linker attachment
- Stable
  - in circulation
  - in lysosomes
- Defined mechanism of action
- Local bystander effect?

Chapter Three Challenges for future research development (future prospect)

As we mentioned above, to bring about the most desirable effects, we must ensure the three components of ADC are well-chosen. In addition, the selection of clinically relevant targets and the position and number of linkages have also been the key determinants of ADC efficacy. So these are exactly what researchers are endeavored to do now.

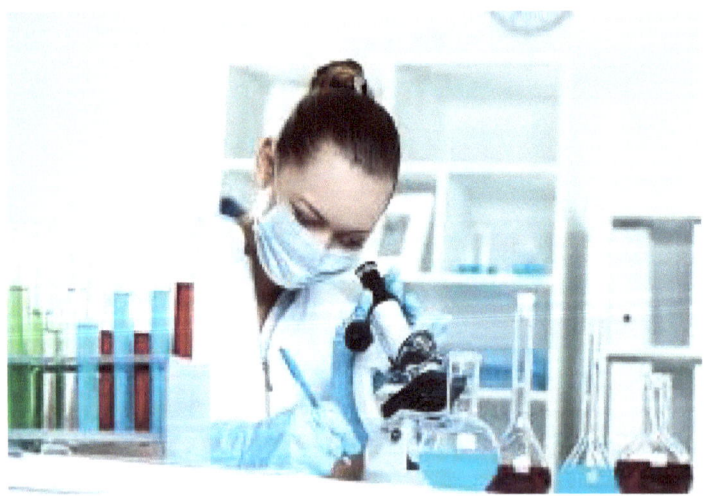

Despite the fact that initially only two ADCs--brentuximab vedotin and trastuzumab emtansine (T-DM1)--have been approved by FDA to enter the market, considerable progress has been achieved in the past few decades, like higher levels of cytotoxic drug conjugation, lower levels of naked antibodies and more-stable linkers between the drug and the antibody. By learning lessons from failures, stresses are now laid on the following aspects:

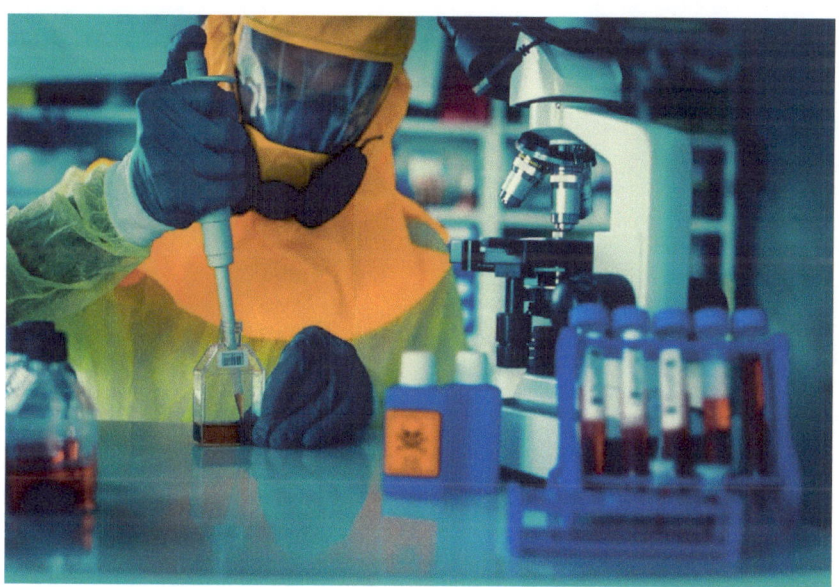

- strategies to select the best target antigens as well as suitable cytotoxic drugs;
- the design of optimized linkers;
- the discovery of bio-orthogonal conjugation chemistries;
- and toxicity issues.

Also, the selection and engineering of antibodies for site-specific drug conjugation, accompanied by the quest for new conjugation chemistries and mechanisms of action, are among top priorities in ADC research as they will contribute to increased stability and higher homogeneity.

Chapter Four Summary

Previously we wandered through a journey about ADC through exploring its definition, main characteristics, mechanism of action (MOA) as well as challenges for future research development. Now it seems perfect time to make a summary as we're almost approaching the end of this article.

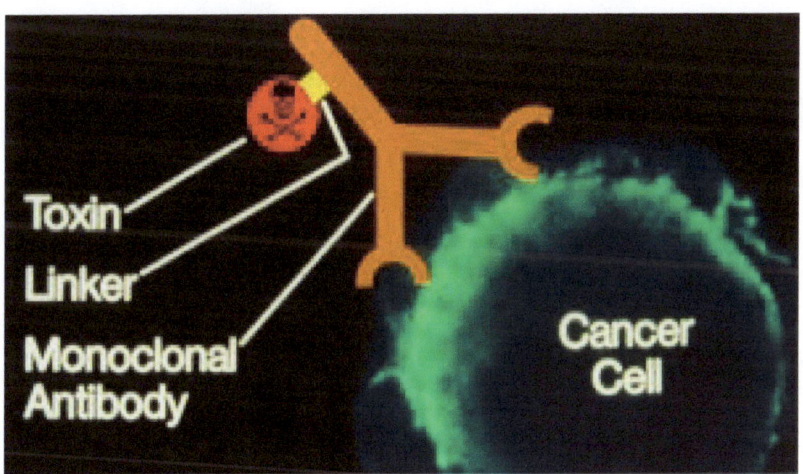

ADC is unquestionably a very promising new cancer treatment loaded with people's hope and ambition to conquer the formidable disease—cancer. Yet, major hurdles still remain there, waiting to be solved, to name just a few: low delivery efficiency, target antigens expressed in normal tissues, the heterogeneity of target antigen expression in the tumour, etc. Surely we are not intimidated at all. So long as more researches are conducted to tackle these issues, so long as target selection has been improved, cytotoxin potency has been enhanced, innovative linkers has been found and drug resistance has been overcome, we are confident that ADCs are very likely to proudly claim its share in the future targeted cancer therapeutics.

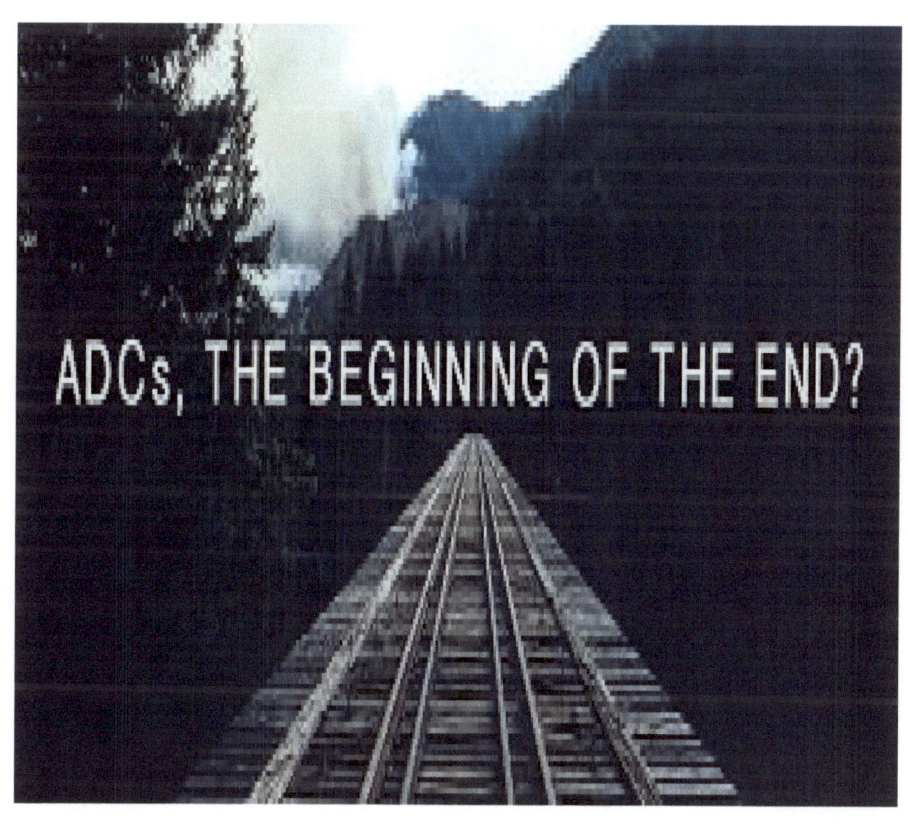

References

https://link.springer.com/chapter/10.1007%2F978-3-319-13081-1_1

https://www.ncbi.nlm.nih.gov/pmc/articles/PMC4613712/

https://adcreview.com/adc-university/adcs-101/antibody-drug-conjugates-adcs/

https://www.ncbi.nlm.nih.gov/pubmed/20025606

https://www.cancer.org/treatment/treatments-and-side-effects/treatment-types/immunotherapy/monoclonal-antibodies.html

http://www.bocsci.com/blog/index.php/antibody-drug-conjugates/

https://www.nature.com/nrd/journal/v16/n5/full/nrd.2016.268.html

http://www.bocsci.com/antibody-drug-conjugates-services.html

www.ingramcontent.com/pod-product-compliance
Lightning Source LLC
Chambersburg PA
CBHW041945240526
45473CB00033B/608